Preventing

HOT-CAR

Deaths

Techniques and Methods

That Work

A handy guide for caregivers

By

G.A. HICKS

Dedication:

To the 44 children who died of heatstroke in the
United States in 2013. Here is praying the
information contained in this guide will have a
positive impact and save many lives that would
have otherwise been lost.

Effective

Solutions

That

Will

Work

For

You

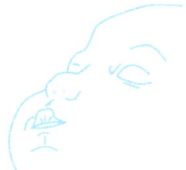

Where We Are Today

Forty-four children died of heatstroke inside of cars last year. These tragic occurrences have come to be known as 'hot-car' deaths. The number one reason given by caregivers as to why this happened was they were distracted and forgot to remove their child from the vehicle, upon reaching their destination.

These are terrible tragedies and each instance raises questions as to how it happened and how these incidents could have been avoided. Many solutions have been offered from updating technology inside of cars, to using manual items as a trigger to help caregivers remember. While we live very busy lives, multitasking and prioritizing, even as we are driving, it is imperative that we keep the presence of our child to the forefront of our mind as we go about our duties.

This guide will ensure you are armed with the techniques and methods that can be used to make 'hot- car' death statistics unfortunate markers from the past.

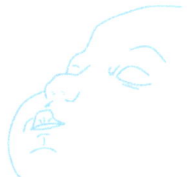

How This Guide Can Help

Preventing Hot-Car Deaths helps by providing techniques that are very clear and will outline how, if you put these methods into action, it will not be possible to forget and leave your child behind in a car.

The techniques will not only help you to accomplish this goal but while performing them, you may find health benefits that may come from doing them. Does this sound odd? Well, keep reading!

Also included at the end of this booklet, are tips and facts about recognizing and preventing heatstroke in children. This additional information will be invaluable in your efforts to improve your safety regiments.

And so, here is to ensuring the statistic for 'hot-car' deaths are '0' at the end of 2015 and each year thereafter.

Technique #1

Talk
To
Me

Talk To Me

The first technique is called *Talk To Me*. Talk to the baby out loud as soon as you get into the car. That is it. They are a person, albeit a little one, after all and talking to them away from the distractions of everyday activities, is a great time for a little one-on-one with them. I have done this since the very beginning of my little girl's life and although I know she did not understand anything I was saying, as soon as we were in the car, I began chatting conversationally. I would ask her how she was doing and tell her where we were going and who we were going to see. I would glance in the rear view mirror and note her many drooling expressions. This glancing in the rear now and again created a very helpful habit.

If we were on the way to the day care, I would talk to her about the things I hoped she would learn and then I would tell her to have a wonderful day and not to fret at naptime. I would tell her I couldn't wait until she met her uncle and aunts, and how they sent their love. There were times when she would make sounds or coo as if to respond and then there were times when there was silence. But in all of my talking, I knew that I wasn't talking to myself but to the little one behind me, even if she couldn't understand me or reply. My voice would sooth and comfort her and this was a nice bond between us. It always felt wonderful talking to her, knowing she was taking in the sound of my voice and inflections and the love and attention I was sending her way. Summer is now three years old and to this day, she is very communicative with me.

My little girl was born with special needs and I feel confident that the talking I have done to her since birth has significantly assisted in her auditory skills and comprehension. Her speech therapist says that she now comprehends at a high level; higher than one would expect of someone with her limitations. I give much of the credit for that to the many hours I spent chatting with her as we went to the museum, shopping, church, library and many other places. Using the *Talk* technique cleared away distractions from my mind and I was able to chat out loud and focus on the present moments with my child and discuss with her the activities we were going to be involved in. The unexpected benefit of aiding in her auditory skills was an added benefit along the way.

Technique #2

Sing

Out

Loud

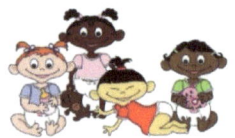

Sing Out Loud

The second technique is called *Sing Out Loud.* Sing childhood songs to your child, out loud, while with him. This can be a great reminder that he is there. I have used this technique on my child since her birth and at this point she sings along with me and we have a grand time of it. Whether you sing with the great voice of Ms. Celia Cruz, or Sir Elton John, or with a voice that you feel should only be heard in the privacy of your shower, by you alone, does not matter. Singing to the child simply reminds you that he is with you. They *love* the sound of your voice and are usually ecstatic when receiving this attention. This may be simple, but it is very effective.

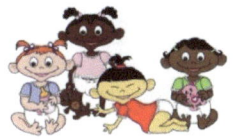

Fun Times...

This is especially fun if you sing nursery rhymes out loud, because why else would you be belting out nursery rhymes verbosely, alone in the car, if not for the little one sitting quietly behind you?

De-stressor...

Studies have shown that singing leads to increases in Cortisol in the brain due to its positive effect on the body. This is beneficial because it is akin to receiving a sedative for stressors that happen in our brain. Driving can be stressful at times and dropping the baby at the child care and getting to work on time is also high on

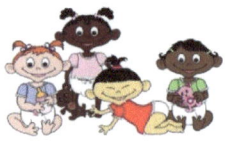

the stress-factor radar. Since this time in the car is a necessary link in our lives to point B, then it can be used in reverse, as a de-stressor and an opportunity for more quality child time; instead of perhaps raising our blood pressure while we think about the next bill, meeting or problem that may be around the corner. Those are the very things that may cause our minds to become *distracted* and overwhelmed and lead to forgetfulness.

Mood regulator…

There will be times when you are not in the 'singing' mood but, being a singer, I can attest to the fact that once you start, you will feel better overall. As a mood regulator singing sooths and calms your mind. In the end, the benefits of singing far outweigh any hesitations that may come about.

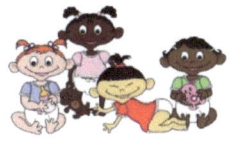

The Little Receptors...

Children are receptive to all that we expose them to and so in the end talking and singing to them can only be positive aspects in many avenues to their development and emotional well being. Many of us lead very busy lives, being distracted by phone calls, texts, multitasking and juggling along the way and sometimes we do not get enough quality time with our little ones. It is better to keep our child to the forefront of our mind by talking or singing to them than to fill the driving time with our thoughts in numerous other places, risking forgetfulness and worst.

Driving to our daily routines, with our child in the rear can be a great way to just stop, take a deep breath and talk to our child or to sing a song to them. It can lessen their crying or fretting time. It can assist them in understanding the inflections and phonetics of language and tone. As well, it is beneficial in bonding with the child, at a time when we may otherwise be preoccupied with stressing.   All of these are benefits to a classic solution.

Forethought

*

Preventing
Heatstroke

*

Safety Tips

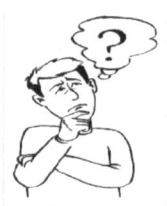

THE POWER

OF

FORETHOUGHT

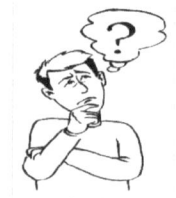

THE POWER OF *FORETHOUGHT*

It is important to know that no matter how much of a hurry we are in, the consequences of forgetting the child is in the car are irreversible. This guide has covered two very effective techniques for ensuring this does not happen.

The remaining pages in this guide focuses on providing information on how to help you recognize the signs of overheating in a child and prevention information; such as the fact that children can become overheated in a car even when it is sitting in the shade. They are not little adults and the difference is significant with respect to their body temperature.

This guide ends with very practical tips from government and private sources that will be useful in your efforts to ensure that your child remains safe and they will help you to better appreciate the value of forethought.

HEATSTROKE

Never leave your child alone in a car for any reason, even with the windows rolled down, or in the shade, or with the air condition on. Children's body temperature can heat up 3 to 5 times faster than adults and so no chances should be taken in this regard. It is not worth the risk. There are never too many habits we can have in place to ensure the safety of our children and we will be well guided to add as many safety regiments as are necessary to our everyday life.

- In 2013, 44 children died of heatstroke in the United States

- Heatstroke begins when the core body temperature reaches about 104 degrees and the thermoregulatory system is overwhelmed. A core temperature of about 107 is lethal.

- Heatstroke fatalities have occurred even in vehicles parked in shaded areas and when the air temperatures where 70 degrees F or less.

Physical Signs of Heatstroke

- Red, hot and moist or dry skin

- No sweating

- A strong rapid pulse or slow weak pulse

- A throbbing headache

- Dizziness

- Nausea

- Confusion

- Behaving grouchy, irritable or acting strangely (out of the ordinary)

Practical SafetyTips

Additional tips are outlined below and they are very simple and practical and you can add them to your daily regiment to ensure additional safety measures are met.

- Never leave a child alone in a car, even if for a few minutes, and even if the air conditioning is on.

- Place an item that you keep on your person, like a briefcase in the backseat so that you will always check the back seat before you leave the car.

- Opening windows will not prevent heatstroke.

- Check with the caregiver after they drop the child off to make sure they didn't forget.

<u>More Safety Tips</u>

- Have daycare call you if your child does not show up.

- Write a note and place it on the dashboard of the car.

- Set a reminder on your cell phone or calendar.

- Keep a stuffed animal in your child's car seat when it is empty and place it in the front seat as a reminder that your child is in the back seat.

- Create a habit to **always** look in both the front and back of the vehicle before locking the door and walking away. **ALWAYS.**

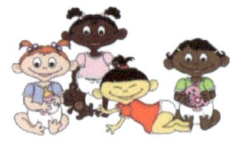

And so…

We live very busy, demanding lives which pull our attention into several directions at once. Our children are our greatest possessions and primary priority and in the end, we will do anything that it takes to ensure their safety. Following the techniques of *Talk To Me* and *Sing Out Loud*, while transporting your child can prove very effective in ensuring that you always remember that your most precious possession is there with you, as well as assisting in lowering your stress level. The other practical tips are also very supportive in helping. In the end, your child is sitting behind you in their car seat, hearing your voice as you sing or talk to him, hanging on to your every word.

Now, who wouldn't want such an attentive audience as that? With your conversation and songs, calming your spirit and lifting theirs, the end of the ride can only end with you exiting the car, turning around, and **remembering** to reach into the back seat for the precious package in the rear.

Hello baby, *we're here*!

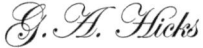

Helpful Hint:

KEEP A COPY OF
THIS BOOK
IN THE
FRONT
AREA OF YOUR CAR

Author

G.A. Hicks is the founder and CEO of Summer's Place of Refuge, a nonprofit group whose mission is to ensure children with developmental and learning disabilities receive education in an environment that uplifts, motivates and challenge minds. Other works by Ms. Hicks include fiction for children and Christian literature. Author may be contacted at the following email address.

Summersplaceofrefuge@gmail.com

Notes:

1. Emily Saarman, *Symposium looks at therapeutic benefits of musical rhythm,* (Stanford, California, 2006)
2. G. Kreutz, U.S. National Library of Medicine, National Institute of Health,*Effects of choir singing or listening on secretory immunoglobulin A, cortisol, and emotional state* (Frankfurt, Germany, 2004)
3. Safercar.gov, Parents Central, *Heatstroke* (2014)